HEALED

*How I Naturally Cured Ulcerative Colitis
Using the Life-Changing Fab Five Protocol*

Table of Contents

Introduction: My Personal Experience with Ulcerative Colitis

Genesis

I woke up one morning with severe cramps and pain in my stomach. It happened around June 2011. I was 32 years old, and my newborn baby was just three months old at that time. I initially thought I had eaten something that did not sit well with my stomach. I believed that with some on-the-shelf tummy medication, it would soon be over. Alas, I was very wrong.

It continued for about a week. I will double up in pain, clutching my stomach; I can barely stand upright. I began to open my bowels several times a day as opposed to the usual "once a day". I could no longer keep anything down. As soon as I ate anything, even just a drink of water, I felt the urgent need to open my bowels.

One day after opening my bowel, I peered at the toilet bowl, and I saw fresh blood in my poop. I was so alarmed that I jumped off the toilet seat in fright. It was just the beginning.

My symptoms had now gone on for two months, and by this time, I had started to lose weight fast. My eyes became sunken, and I grew weaker and weaker with each passing day. I had gone from a size 12 UK to a size 8 UK. My clothes were beginning to hang on my body, and people started to notice and comment on my sudden weight loss. I became so afraid to eat or drink anything because each time I tried, it triggered severe tummy cramps, which would force me back to the loo to pass it out. I started passing out more and more blood. The scariest part for me was that I was beginning to lose control of my bowels. I had to be on the toilet seat just a few seconds after the cramps started. Otherwise, I would soil myself! At this point, I realised I needed to seek medical attention.

Diagnosis

My doctor told me I needed a test to see what was happening in my stomach. He said they would focus on my colon, where waste was passing out.

I underwent a procedure called a colonoscopy, a long flexible tube with a camera at the tip that passed from my anus into my colon. It was quite a painful and uncomfortable procedure.

The test result showed that my colon was severely inflamed and bleeding, and this was the primary cause of everything I had been experiencing.

Precisely in November 2011, I was diagnosed with Ulcerative Colitis. A medical term for "Ulcer in the colon". A lifelong disease with no known cure! My doctor said there was no known cause for this disease so far, and one of the possible contributing factors could be "Stress".

He said they were going to manage the ailment by placing me on medication permanently. I felt shattered!

Conventional Treatments Received

First, I was placed on steroids for two months to calm all the craziness in my colon. They advised me to immediately stop breastfeeding my 6-month-old baby because the medication could have side effects on him. Hearing this made me so miserable.

The steroids worked well and reduced the severe cramps, but I was still opening my bowels several times a day. After those two months, I was taken off the steroids and prescribed my primary medication.

i. **Mezavant XL**: a sizable tablet, four per day in the morning, which will slowly release throughout the day to calm my symptoms.

ii. **Ferrous Fumarate 210mg** per day: small iron tablets to reinstate the iron level in my body and manage my severe anaemia, which I had developed due to so much blood loss

iii. **Dicyclomine 10mg**- a small tablet for my cramps.

Motivation for seeking natural remedies.

I accepted my fate and focused on taking my medication with the hope of managing my disease well.

Over the next couple of years, the medication helped manage my ailment. The cramps reduced drastically, and I opened my bowels less often; the bleeding also reduced, and I gained back control of my bowels.

But I observed so many foods and drinks that I could no longer tolerate - Any food and beverages containing gluten, sugar, flour, dairy products, fried foods, oil, fizzy drinks, cereal, spice or spicy food, popcorn, and more! I could not even tolerate healthy stuff like fruits and vegetables! My favourite fruits, bananas and watermelon, had become a no-go area. If I attempted to eat or drink any of this, I would return to square one! Suffering severe flare-ups, and all of the initial symptoms will be back! (Severe cramps, bleeding, diarrhoea, and loss of my bowel.) despite using my medication.

The only drinks that I could tolerate were water and green tea, nothing else.

The only food that sat well was gluten-free oats eaten plain, plain boiled rice, boiled egg, and plain chicken breast. I had to stick to this for the next four years! What a Life!

I also continued routine colonoscopy checks. The inflammation remained there. Each time, they would extract polyps from the wall of my colon to test and see if they had not become cancerous. That was the biggest fright! They told me that cancer could quickly grow on the inflamed parts of my colon. They also said as with any conventional medication, long-term use could result in severe side effects. The longer I used this medication, the more worried I became.

My lifestyle changed; I lost confidence and became a shadow of myself. I could barely go out and socialise because I could not eat what everybody was eating; hence, my social life suffered' I didn't want to risk eating something that might trigger a flare-up, causing me to lose control of my bowel, soil myself, and feel embarrassed. Whenever I went out, I would join people and eat nothing.

I started wearing pampers to manage any mishaps. I also ensured to be in environments where I could access the toilers quickly and easily.

I became sad, depressed, and very malnourished because I was not getting enough nutrients or a balanced diet. My anaemia stayed on despite taking iron tablets every single day. I was a weak, fragile version of myself. All this made me realise I could not continue living this way. After four years, I started researching how to heal this ailment naturally. I did not want to be stuck on conventional medication for the rest of my life. It was not even curing me anyway! Hence, I began my journey towards natural healing.

After trying out so many natural options, I eventually found a combination of 5 natural foods and supplements that cured me of Ulcerative Colitis!

THE BOOK'S OBJECTIVES

- To offer hope and practical advice for others who have ulcerative Colitis.
- I want to share all the facts I learned about ulcerative Colitis during my research, which includes:
- Better understanding of Ulcerative Colitis
- The impact that Stress has on this condition and stress management techniques,
- I want to share the five natural food combinations that led to my complete cure and provide advice on how I use them daily. I believe this will help someone also find healing.

DISCLAIMER: The content presented in this book:

HEALED

How I Naturally Cured Ulcerative Colitis Using the Life-Changing Fab Five Protocol

is based on my experiences and is intended for educational purposes only. I am not a healthcare professional so the methods discussed should not be viewed as advice or a replacement for professional diagnosis and treatment.

Ulcerative colitis is a health condition. It is crucial to consult with a qualified healthcare provider before implementing any new treatments, supplements or lifestyle changes. What worked for me may not be suitable for everyone as individual results can vary.

This book aims to offer guidance than personalized medical care. The author and publisher are not liable for any effects or outcomes resulting from following the suggestions, preparations or procedures outlined in this book.

Always seek guidance from your doctor or another qualified healthcare provider if you have any concerns, about your health or specific medical conditions. It's important not to disregard advice or delay seeking it based on information found in this book.

1

Getting to Know
Ulcerative Colitis

Definition of Ulcerative Colitis

Ulcerative colitis (UC) is a bowel disease that causes inflammation and ulcers in the digestive system. It mainly impacts the lining of the intestine (colon) and rectum. Having a grasp of this condition is vital for discovering natural ways to manage and potentially treat it. This chapter will delve into the signs, reasons, risk factors and traditional treatments for colitis laying the groundwork for the natural approaches discussed later in this book.

Signs of Ulcerative Colitis

Ulcerative colitis can manifest symptoms that vary in intensity and frequency. Common signs are:

1. **Stomach Pain and Cramping**: discomfort often centred in the abdomen is a key feature of UC. This discomfort typically comes with cramping.

2. **Bowel Issues**: Frequent episodes of bowel movements with blood or pus are common symptoms. The seriousness can range from mild to severe.

3. **Bleeding from Rectum**: The presence of blood in stool or rectal bleeding is an indicator of UC. It can be unsettling and is a primary aspect of the condition.

4. **Unintended Weight Loss**: Involuntary weight loss may happen due to constant stooling and decreased appetite.

5. **Fatigue:** lasting tiredness and a general sense of feeling unwell can result from inflammation and anaemia.

6. **Fever:** Sometimes, a slight fever may be present, indicating inflammation. The symptoms may vary between periods of worsening and improvement. During these times, the symptoms might completely disappear, only to come back later.

Causes of Ulcerative Colitis

The exact cause of colitis is still unknown. However, it is believed that several factors play a role in its development.

1. **Immune System Response**: Ulcerative colitis is believed to involve a response where the immune system mistakenly attacks the cells in the colon, thinking they are harmful invaders. This results in inflammation.

2. **Genetic Predisposition**: Having a family history of colitis or other inflammatory bowel diseases increases the risk. Certain genetic traits have been associated with a likelihood of developing colitis.

3. **Environmental Factors**: Aspects such as diet, pollution, and lifestyle choices may impact the onset and progression of colitis. These factors can interact with predispositions to trigger the disease.

Risk Factors.

Recognising the risk factors for colitis can aid in detection and management.

- UC commonly starts before the age of 30. It can also occur at any stage of life. Another peak in the number of cases is observed in individuals between the ages of 50 and 70.
- A family history of UC or other inflammatory bowel diseases raises the risk factor for an individual.
- People with ancestry are more prone to developing UC, although it can affect individuals from any ethnic background.
- Higher rates of UC are documented in developed nations, urban regions and colder climates.
- Traditional medical interventions focus on reducing inflammation, managing symptoms and achieving remission. These treatments encompass:

Medications

Aminosalicylates: These anti-inflammatory medications are typically used as the treatment for moderate UC.

Corticosteroids: Employed for short-term management during flare-ups, these potent anti-inflammatory drugs come with significant side effects when used long-term.

Immunomodulators: These drugs assist in altering the system's response to reduce inflammation.

Biologics: Targeted treatments that hinder components of the immune response. In situations where other treatments are ineffective, surgery to remove the colon (colectomy) may be required. While this can offer a solution for the condition it also brings its set of challenges and adjustments to one's lifestyle.

Although not a remedy, making dietary changes and practising stress management techniques can help in symptom control and enhance overall quality of life.

Moving Forward, the initial step towards managing and overcoming colitis involves understanding the condition. By identifying the symptoms, causes and risk factors and familiarizing oneself with treatments, individuals can make choices about their well-being. Many individuals are now exploring methods to manage and potentially treat UC aiming for side effects and a more holistic approach to health. The following sections of this book will discuss these approaches in detail, including modifications, natural food remedies, stress management strategies and lifestyle changes that have proven beneficial for many in finding relief and achieving long-term remission.

Embarking on your journey towards a remedy for colitis begins with knowledge. With this awareness at hand, you are prepared to explore approaches that empower you to take charge of your health and wellness.

2

Healthy Eating and Nutrition

When I started my journey to treat colitis changing my diet was a game changer. Understanding how food impacted my body was key to managing and eventually overcoming my condition. In this chapter, I'll discuss the crucial adjustments in my healing journey, such as the foods I embraced and those I avoided. Additionally, I'll touch on the guiding principles and beliefs that shaped my nutrition decisions.

Exploring the Gut Health Relationship

The gut is home to trillions of bacteria, forming an ecosystem known as the gut microbiome. This microbiome plays a role in digestion, immunity and overall well-being. For individuals with colitis, maintaining a balanced gut microbiome is crucial as it can impact inflammation and immune function.

Foods that Trigger Inflammation to Stay Away From

There are some certain types of foods and beverages that can worsen inflammation and ulcerative colitis symptoms. Here are the key types of foods that I found important to steer of:

Processed Foods: These items are often loaded with preservatives, artificial additives and unhealthy fats that can spark inflammation. This category includes packaged snacks, fast food items and pre-packaged meals.

Dairy Products: Individuals with colitis experience lactose intolerance, making it challenging to digest dairy products. I found that cutting back on dairy helped me avoid discomfort.

Gluten: A protein in wheat, barley and rye, can trigger inflammation in people especially those with celiac disease or gluten sensitivity. I discovered that removing gluten from my diet significantly improved my symptoms.

Sugary Foods and Beverages: Excessive sugar consumption can disrupt the guts balance. Lead to inflammation. This includes treats, desserts, soft drinks and some fruit juices.

Alcohol and Caffeine: Both alcohol and caffeine can irritate the tract and worsen symptoms. Limiting or removing these items from my diet proved helpful in managing flare ups.

Embracing Anti-Inflammatory Foods

To support healing, I focused on incorporating foods that enhance gut health and reduce inflammation. Here are the main elements of my inflammatory eating plan:

(It is important to mention that I could only tolerate most of the below-mentioned foods after my healing from the "FAB FIVE" had started- to be discussed in the next chapter)

Fruits and Vegetables: Fresh organic fruits and vegetables are packed with essential vitamins, minerals and antioxidants. Some beneficial choices include berries, leafy greens, carrots and squash. These foods provided nutrients while being gentle on my system.

Lean Proteins: Protein is crucial, for repairing tissues and supporting the system. I included sources like fish, chicken and plant-based proteins such as beans and lentils. These protein options are easier on the stomach compared to meat and other fatty meats.

Healthy Fats: Omega 3 fatty acids found in fish, flaxseeds and walnuts have inflammatory properties. I also added avocados, olive oil and coconut oil for their fats.

Gluten-free grains: I opted for free alternatives like quinoa, brown rice and oats. These grains provided fibre without causing inflammation.

Fermented Foods: Options like yoghurt (dairy versions), kefir, sauerkraut and kimchi are packed with probiotics that promote a gut microbiome. Including these foods helped rebalance the bacteria in my gut.

Herbs and Spices; Certain herbs and spices boast inflammatory properties. Turmeric, ginger, garlic and cinnamon became meal's ingredients, enhancing both flavour and health benefits.

Meal Planning and Mindful Eating

Embarking on a regimen requires careful planning and mindfulness.

Here are a few things I did to keep myself on the path:

1. **Meal Preparation**: Getting my meals ready in advance, ensured that I always had choices at hand, cutting down on the urge to opt for snacks or quick meals.
2. **Balanced Eating**: Each meal consisted of a mix of protein, good fats and carbohydrates to maintain energy levels and aid digestion.
3. **Staying Hydrated:** Keeping up with water intake was crucial for well-being. It helped my digestive system function smoothly.

Herbal teas like green tea, chamomile, ginger or peppermint tea also provide support for digestion.

4. **Tuning into My Body**: Being mindful of how my body responds to foods helped me adjust my diet. I maintained a food diary to monitor what I consumed and its impact on my well-being.

Supplements and Natural Solutions

Alongside adjustments, specific supplements and natural remedies played a role in supporting my recovery:

1. Probiotics: Adding top-quality probiotics helped in restoring and maintaining a gut microbiome.
2. Omega 3 Supplements; Introducing fish oil or flaxseed oil supplements offered inflammatory advantages.
3. Aloe Vera Juice: Renowned for its calming properties aloe vera juice aided in reducing inflammation and promoting healing within the GI tract.

Bone broth, which is packed with collagen and amino acids has been found to promote gut healing and enhance health.

Personalised Approach

It's crucial to understand that what may be effective for one person might not yield the results for another. Everyone's experience with colitis is unique. Discovering the most suitable dietary approach can be a journey that requires time and patience. Seeking guidance from healthcare professionals like nutritionists or gastroenterologists can offer tailored advice and assistance.

Conclusion

In my experience, diet and nutrition played a role in my natural healing journey from ulcerative colitis. By eliminating some foods, embracing gut choices and being attuned to my body's requirements, I created an environment conducive to healing while minimising flare-ups. Remember, the path to wellness is individualised, with finding the right dietary balance being crucial in managing and overcoming colitis. In the following section, we will delve into the significance of lifestyle adjustments, such as stress management and physical activity, in supporting health and well-being.

3

Healing Power of the "Fab Five"- The Natural Remedies and Supplements that Cured Me

Exploring the Benefits of the "FAB Five" for Ulcerative Colitis Treatment and Incorporating Them into My Everyday Diet Routine

During my journey to treat Colitis naturally, I conducted extensive research over a couple of months, trying out many natural foods and supplements that I found to have anti-inflammatory properties.

Then, I came across the healing properties of a combination of five natural Foods and Supplements.

These remedies played a role in my healing process, offering benefits that worked together harmoniously to restore my gut health. In this Chapter, I will delve into my experiences and the profound impact that **soursop, flaxseed, honey, black seed oil,** and **probiotics** had on my path to well-being and complete recovery. I affectionately refer to them as the "FAB FIVE"!

1. Soursop

The Superfruit Packed with Nutrients

Soursop, or Graviola or Guanabana, is a fruit celebrated for its rich composition and potential health advantages. This green fruit with spiky skin contains various vitamins, minerals, and antioxidants that can aid in reducing inflammation and supporting gut health.

Advantages for Ulcerative Colitis

Anti-Inflammatory Properties: Soursop is abundant in inflammatory compounds that can assist in alleviating gut inflammation typical in ulcerative colitis patients.

Rich in antioxidants: Soursop's antioxidants help combat stress levels that usually heighten during inflammation.

Supporting Gut Health: Soursop is rich in fibre, which helps with digestion and keeping your bowel movements regular, which is essential for managing ulcerative Colitis.

Ways to Enjoy Soursop

I like to include soursop in my meals by eating the fruit, blending it into smoothies, or enjoying soursop tea. It's essential to remember that while soursop has its benefits, it's best to consume it in moderation due to its effects.

2. Flaxseed

A Nutrient-Rich Seed

Flaxseed, a brown seed, is packed with omega-3 fatty acids, fibre, and lignans. It has been valued for centuries for its health advantages in supporting digestive wellness.

Advantages for Ulcerative Colitis

Anti-Inflammatory Properties: The omega-3 fatty acids in flaxseeds possess inflammatory qualities that help calm the inflamed intestinal lining associated with ulcerative Colitis.

Fiber Rich: Flaxseed is a source of insoluble fibres that promote regular bowel movements and overall digestive well-being.

Healing Lignans: These natural compounds have inflammatory attributes contributing to gut healing processes.

Incorporating Flaxseed into Your Diet

I've discovered that mixing ground flaxseed into my smoothies' oatmeal, and salads is a way to include it in my meals. Remember to use ground flaxseed rather than seeds for better nutrient absorption.

Tip: Another excellent source of omega-3 three fatty acids is **OMEGA 3 FATTY ACID FISH OIL Supplements. (Holland and Barrett)** I take one tablet per day. Especially sometimes when I am unable to have my flaxseed during the day. **(Check out tips for recommended brands, daily intake, and usage suggestions in the Appendices section)**

3. Organic honey

Serves as more than a sweetener; it also acts as a potent remedy with various health advantages. Its antibacterial, anti-inflammatory and antioxidant qualities make it a beneficial supplement for individuals with Colitis.

Advantages for Ulcerative Colitis

Soothing Qualities: Honey can relieve the system, lessening irritation and discomfort linked to Colitis.

Antibacterial Benefits: Its innate antibacterial attributes can help ward off infections that may worsen colitis symptoms.

Supports Healing: The antioxidants present in honey assist in the restoration of the lining and fostering gut well-being.

Incorporating Organic Honey

I use organic honey as a natural sweetener in my oatmeal, tea, smoothies, and kefir. Opting for quality organic honey is essential to reap the full benefits.

4. Black Seed Oil:

An Ancient Elixir tagged "The Blessed Seed".

Black seed oil, extracted from Nigella sativa seeds, has been revered in medicine for centuries. Dubbed "the cure for everything except death "black seed oil boasts an array of health rewards.

Advantages for Ulcerative Colitis

Potent Anti-Inflammatory Properties: Black seed oil possesses inflammatory characteristics that can aid in reducing colon inflammation associated with ulcerative Colitis.

Support for the Immune System: Black seed oil assists in regulating the system, which is vital for managing conditions such as ulcerative Colitis.

Promoting Digestive Health: Using black seed oil can enhance digestion and alleviate issues like bloating and gas.

Incorporating Black Seed Oil into Your Routine

Out of the FAB FIVE," Black seed oil was the only one I could not tolerate the taste. The oil left a funny aftertaste in my mouth. Then I discovered and tried the capsule version (Blackseed Oil Capsules- one daily which I later increased to two), which could be swallowed immediately with water without tasting the oil itself. That worked for me!

The one I use is from www.theblessedseed.com**(The Blessed Seed Strong Black Seed Oil (halal Gelatine) Capsules)**

(Check out tips for recommended brands, daily intake, and usage suggestions in the Appendices section)

5. Probiotics

Probiotics consist of bacteria and yeasts that are beneficial for maintaining gut health. They are essential for preserving gut flora balance for individuals dealing with ulcerative Colitis.

Advantages for Ulcerative Colitis

Restoring Gut Equilibrium: Probiotics aid reinstating the balance of gut bacteria that may be disrupted in cases of Colitis.

Alleviating Inflammation: By encouraging a response, probiotics can help reduce inflammation within the gut.

Enhancing Digestive Function: Probiotics boost digestion and nutrient absorption, addressing challenges faced by colitis patients.

Integrating Probiotics into Your Diet

I included high-quality probiotics Supplements. This comes from capsules, which can be purchased on the shelf from health stores. The one I use is from Holland and Barrett **(PROBIO 7. ORIGINAL-10 BILLION FRIENDLY BACTERIA)- (Check out tips for recommended brands, daily intake, and usage suggestions in the Appendices section)**

I also incorporated naturally occurring probiotics in my meals through fermented foods, the one that works well with my stomach is kefir.

My Breakthrough

In wrapping up, the natural foods and supplement treatments I used were crucial in helping me recover from Colitis. **Soursop, flaxseed honey, black seed oil,** and **probiotics** each provided benefits that aided the elimination of inflammation, supporting gut healing and improving overall digestive health. By incorporating these remedies into my routine, I experienced complete healing and a better quality of life.

All the significant symptoms of Colitis disappeared after about two months of consistently using the "FAB FIVE".

This change happened to me by the end of 2019. During this time, I continued using my conventional prescription. I was eager to share the good news with my doctor.

However, the lockdown happened in 2020, and because I was terrified of attending the hospital for my routine blood check (I needed this to receive my medication continuously), My prescription supplies stopped for the next two years. These are the medications I had used consistently for eight years, non-stop!

Initially, I was worried about the lack of my prescribed medication, but I continued with the "FAB FIVE", and continued to feel perfect and healed in my gut; I never looked back to conventional treatment since then.

In 2022, I finally got to attend a routine checkup at the hospital. I excitedly shared my news with my doctor, who didn't seem so convinced and said he had to run tests on me, to determine if I was as well as I claimed.

We agreed that I would return to my prescriptions if my inflammation remained active.

The results came, and I was declared to be in remission! My doctor made no further prescriptions.

I was set FREE!

TOP TIPS.

It is essential to note that once I discovered the healing power of THE FAB FIVE,

1. I have continued to incorporate them into all my daily meal plans. (I firmly believe that being consistent with THE FAB FIVE played a significant role in my permanent healing)
2. To ensure consistent use of THE FAB FIVE daily and avoid forgetting, I have them all at breakfast.

(I cook my gluten-free oat and let it cool down a bit. I then mix in my organic honey, soursop smoothie and blended flaxseed. I also added almond milk **containing no sugar** for a better taste. Once I've had my porridge, I then take my probiotic and blackseed oil capsules (I started with one and increased to about six months later)

Finally, it's essential to consult with a healthcare professional before starting any treatment plan to ensure it's safe and suitable for your specific needs. I sincerely hope THE FAB FIVE works for you too!

In the next Chapter, we'll delve into how lifestyle adjustments, such as managing Stress and engaging in activities, have contributed to maintaining my good health and well-being.

4

Coping with Stress

Dealing with "stress" was something I knew I needed to focus on. Reflecting on the timeline leading up to my illness, it was clear that intense stress played a role in triggering the disease.

In the months leading to my diagnosis, I was going through forms of abuse in my marriage. (Domestic, physical and emotional). Also, being left to solely take responsibility for two children, including a newborn, while dealing with pain, fatigue, and constant weakness took its toll.

Realizing that addressing the root cause of my illness, Stress, was essential for any progress, I made the decision to separate from my abuser and move far away from him. This marked the beginning of my healing journey.

My Mum also kindly moved in with me for a good couple of years to assist with caring for my kids. This greatly alleviated a lot of the physical stress I was going through alone. I am eternally grateful to her.

I discovered that stress plays a role in both causing and worsening colitis (UC). As I set out to heal from UC, managing stress became an aspect of my approach. In this section, I will discuss the techniques for handling stress that were instrumental in my recovery. These strategies have not only helped alleviate UC symptoms but also enhanced my overall well-being.

Recognizing the Link Between Stress and UC

Stress has an impact on the system.

When we feel stressed our bodies release stress hormones, like cortisol and adrenaline. These hormones can cause inflammation in the gut, worsening UC symptoms. That's why it's important to learn how to manage stress if you want to handle or even heal UC naturally.

Practicing Mindfulness Meditation

I came across a tool called mindfulness meditation. It involves focusing on the moment and observing thoughts and sensations without judgment. Here's how you can incorporate meditation into your routine:

1. **Make Time**: Set aside 10 to 20 minutes every day for meditation in a quiet space where you can be alone.
2. **Get Comfortable**: Sit or lie down in a position, close your eyes and take some breaths.
3. **Focus on Your Breathing**: Concentrate on your breath feeling the air come in and go out through your nostrils.
4. **Acknowledge Your Thoughts**: When thoughts pop up recognise them. Gently redirect your attention back to your breathing.
5. **Stay Consistent**: Practice daily to feel the effects over time.

Deep Breathing Exercises

Deep breathing exercises are an effective way to alleviate stress by triggering the body's relaxation response, which lowers heart rate and blood pressure.

One method that has been helpful for me is as follows:

1. Get comfortable; Find a position, either sitting or lying down and place your hands on your belly.

2. Take a breath; Inhale through your nose, letting your belly rise as you fill up your lungs.

3. Hold it in; Pause for a moment.

4. Exhale gently; Release the air through your mouth, allowing your belly to fall.

5. Repeat this process; Keep up this cycle for about 5 to 10 minutes.

Staying active physically

Engaging in activities is an effective way to handle stress. Exercise triggers the release of endorphins which are natural mood boosters. It also helps reduce the levels of stress hormones in the body. Here are some types of activities that I included in my routine.

1. **Yoga:** This practice involves poses, breathing techniques and meditation – great for stress reduction and promoting gut health.

2. **Walking**: A yet exercise that can be done anywhere. Walking amidst nature can be especially soothing.

3. **Strength training**: Building muscle and enhancing well-being, through strength training can help increase confidence levels and alleviate stress.

Eating foods can help stress levels

Here are some tips that I've found to be useful:

1. **Balanced Eating:** Include plenty of fruits, veggies, whole grains, lean proteins and healthy fats, in your diet.

2. **Watch Your Intake**: Try to limit your consumption of caffeine and sugar as they can heighten feelings of anxiety and stress.

3. **Stay Hydrated**; Make sure to drink water throughout the day to keep yourself hydrated.

Sleep Hygiene

The Significance of Quality Sleep

Quality sleep is essential for healing and overall well-being. Poor sleep can weaken the system. Increase stress both of which can worsen UC symptoms. Prioritising sleep habits made a difference in my recovery journey.

Make it a priority to get sleep each night. Aim for 7 to 9 hours of quality sleep to give your body the chance to rest, recover and recharge.

Establishing a Sleep Conducive Atmosphere:

I adjusted my sleeping environment to enhance sleep quality. This involved keeping my bedroom cool, dark and quiet, investing in comfortable mattresses and pillows as well as avoiding electronic devices before bedtime.

Establishing a Nighttime Routine:

Creating a bedtime ritual helped my body recognise that it was time to relax. This involved activities such as reading, taking a bath or doing gentle stretches. I made sure to avoid caffeine and heavy meals in the evening to improve my sleep quality.

Social Support

Having a support system is key in handling stress. Surround yourself with understanding individuals who can offer support during times. Here's how you can establish and nurture a circle:

1. **Seek Help**: Don't hesitate to reach out to friends and family for assistance or talk about how you're feeling.
2. **Connect with Support Groups**: Consider becoming part of a support group for those dealing with UC or chronic illnesses.

3. **Professional Guidanc**e: It's okay to seek help from a therapist or counsellor if you feel it would be beneficial.

Hobbies and Interests

Engaging, in activities that bring you joy can be a way to alleviate stress. Whether it's painting, writing, gardening, playing music, dancing or reading, prioritize hobbies that bring relaxation and happiness into your life.

In wrapping up, it's crucial to handle stress when aiming to heal colitis through natural means. By integrating practices like mindfulness meditation, deep breathing exercises, staying active, journaling, getting rest, eating well, seeking good social connections and engaging in activities you love on a regular basis, you can lower stress levels and enhance your well-being.

Keep in mind that the key is discovering what suits you best and integrating it into your life consistently.

5

Embracing Change in Everyday Life

Throughout my journey towards healing and overcoming Ulcerative Colitis (UC), I gained an understanding of how lifestyle adjustments can impact the management and recovery from this condition. While changes in diet and treatments were aspects of my healing journey, the broader significance of lifestyle modifications cannot be overlooked. This chapter explores the lifestyle changes that played a role in my path to recovery.

Key Points

- Managing Stress (as discussed earlier in Chapter 4)
- Adopting Healthy Eating Habits and Nutrition (as mentioned in Chapter 2)
- Prioritizing Quality Sleep (as highlighted in Chapter 4)
- Incorporating Physical Activity

Regular Physical activity offers numerous benefits for overall well-being and is a valuable tool in managing UC symptoms. It aids digestion, boosts immunity, enhances mood and helps reduce inflammation, which is essential for UC management.

I experimented with forms of exercise to find what worked best for me. Engaging in activities, like walking, swimming and cycling allowed me to maintain a lifestyle without triggering symptoms or worsening my condition.

Maintaining an exercise routine was key. I made sure to set 30 minutes for activity every day.

Listening to Your Body

Paying attention to your body's cues is crucial in adjusting your exercise routine based on how you feel. When faced with flare-ups I discovered that activities, like stretching or yoga provided relief without putting strain on my body.

Building a Support System

Having a network of support is essential when dealing with a health condition like UC. I leaned on my family and friends, and online communities for guidance, encouragement and emotional backing. Sharing experiences with others going through the same challenge brought me comfort and motivation.

Nurturing Relationships

Staying connected with others and engaging in activities played a role in maintaining my outlook. Simple acts like taking walks with friends or having heart to heart conversations with loved ones had an impact on my well-being.

Embracing Positivity and Mental Wellness

Adopting a mindset was key to my healing journey. Practicing gratitude by focusing on the things I was grateful, for each day helped me shift from focusing on hardships to counting my blessings. Whenever needed I did not hesitate to seek help.

Participating in therapy or counselling sessions has provided me with tools to navigate the challenges of living with UC. Attending therapy has truly assisted me in finding ways to cope with my anxiety and maintain a positive outlook.

Implementing these lifestyle changes has had an impact, on how I manage Ulcerative Colitis. By incorporating stress management techniques engaging in activities that promote relaxation establishing a support network and fostering positivity I have created an environment for my healing journey. It is crucial to recognize that each person's journey is unique, so it is essential to find what works best for you and adapt as needed.

6

Maintaining Optimal Health
for the Long Term

When managing colitis naturally it's essential to stay committed, aware and dedicated, to the lifestyle changes that have helped you recover. Achieving remission is a milestone. Sustaining it requires ongoing dedication to maintaining balance and resilience in the face of potential challenges. This chapter provides guidance and strategies on how to preserve your well-being and prevent the recurrence of colitis symptoms.

Here are some key points we've covered previously:

To Do List

Embracing Your New Routine: After overcoming the symptoms and obstacles of colitis, attaining remission can feel like a new beginning. It is important to recognize that adjusting to your new norm involves actively prioritizing your health. This includes monitoring your symptoms, listening to your body's cues and making adaptations along the journey.

Regular Health Checkups: Regular appointments, with a healthcare provider who understands your condition and natural healing process are crucial. These visits help monitor your health status watch for signs of inflammation and ensure the functioning of your system. Periodic blood tests, colonoscopies and other diagnostic tests may be utilized to assess your progress.

Paying Attention to Your Body's Signals: It is important to listen to what your body is telling you. Pay attention to any changes in your digestion, energy levels and overall health. Being aware of these signals can help prevent issues from developing into more serious problems. Keeping a health journal to track your diet, symptoms and any patterns you notice can be helpful.

Taking Care of Your Nutrition: Managing your health and promoting wellness are greatly impacted by the foods you eat. Continuing to follow an anti-inflammatory diet is key. Here are some important things to consider:

Eating a Balanced Diet: Ensure that your meals include a variety of fruits, vegetables, lean proteins, healthy fats and whole grains. This diverse mix will provide your body with nutrients and support overall well-being.

Probiotics and Prebiotics: Incorporate probiotic rich foods into your diet to promote a healthy gut. Foods like yogurt, kefir, sauerkraut and other fermented foods are sources of probiotics. Prebiotics found in foods like garlic, onions and bananas help nourish the bacteria in your gut.

Staying Hydrated: Maintaining hydration is vital, for health. Be sure to drink water throughout the day to keep your system functioning well.

Avoiding Triggers: Keep steering off foods and substances that trigger your symptoms as you have identified them before. Some common triggers, for flare ups include processed foods, sugary treats and specific food additives. Be mindful of your diet especially when experimenting with foods.

Emotional Support and Physical Support: Living with a condition like colitis can be emotionally challenging. It's crucial to address your well-being as part of your health plan.

Staying Informed and Educated: Continue learning about colitis, natural healing methods and general health and wellness. Staying updated on research findings, treatment options and strategies can improve your well-being.

Reading and Research: Delve into books, articles and research studies on colitis and natural health to enhance your knowledge in these areas. Being informed enables you to make decisions about your health journey.

Engaging with Healthcare Providers: It is important to maintain communication with your healthcare team. Share any insights or approaches you come across and discuss how they could complement your healthcare regimen.

Celebrating Milestones: Finally, take a moment to rejoice in the milestones and achievements along the way. Recognize the progress you've made by prioritizing your well-being. Celebrating these wins can boost your motivation.

Acknowledging Achievements: Take a moment to celebrate the progress you have achieved since you were diagnosed. Reflect on the improvements, in your health overall well-being and quality of life.

Setting New Goals: Establish objectives for your health and wellness to continue moving on your journey towards improvement. These goals can encompass fitness, nutrition mental well-being or personal growth.

Maintaining long term health after healing colitis requires a proactive mindset. By staying attentive making choices and prioritizing your well-being you can enjoy a fulfilling life from the constraints of chronic illness. Remember that your health voyage is ongoing and every step you take to uphold your well-being brings you closer to a healthier tomorrow.

Conclusion

Recap, Encouragement, and Gratitude

Embarking on the path to combat Colitis naturally has been a transformative journey. As you finish reading this book, I hope you feel empowered, inspired, and equipped with wisdom to guide you to healing and wellness. Let's pause to reflect on the insights gained and how they can influence your health endeavours.

The Strength of Natural Healing

Throughout this publication, we have delved into the potential of natural healing techniques in managing and curing Colitis. From comprehending the causes of inflammation to adopting modifications, stress management strategies, and holistic approaches, you have discovered that healing goes beyond just treating symptoms—it involves nurturing your body, mind, and soul.

Embracing a Comprehensive Approach

A perspective lies at the core of natural healing initiatives.

Understanding the importance of treating your body and recognising how aspects of your life – such as diet, Stress, emotions, and habits – contribute to your overall well-being is vital. By embracing a rounded lifestyle, you empower yourself to take charge of your health and make decisions that promote lasting healing.

Reaching remission from Colitis is a milestone that requires dedication, persistence, and commitment. Acknowledging the work put in along the way and viewing the journey as an opportunity for growth and self-discovery is crucial. Embrace the lessons learned. The inner strength gained while continuing to prioritise your health.

Remaining Informed and Engaged

From now on, staying informed about healing methods is essential, listening to your body's signals and being willing to adapt when necessary. Your dedication to learning and evolving will be instrumental in sustaining health over time and preventing setbacks.

Fostering Inner Strength

Healing is not a one-time achievement but an ongoing process. As you navigate life's challenges gracefully, building resilience, cultivating patience, and embracing adaptability will be traits.

Remember that facing challenges is a part of life's journey. Each obstacle you encounter provides an opportunity for growth and resilience.

Celebrate your accomplishments no matter how small they may seem. These milestones reflect your work and commitment, reminding you of your progress.

Acknowledging the support you've received from loved ones, healthcare professionals, and community groups is essential. Their presence and assistance have played a role in your healing process.

As you move forward, approach the future with optimism and confidence. Your journey has equipped you with insights and tools to prioritise your well-being. Trust in your knowledge. Strive for a life filled with balance, vitality, and happiness.

Your experience of overcoming Colitis not only highlights the strength of natural healing but also serves as inspiration for others facing similar challenges. Share your story, extend a helping hand to those in need, and be a beacon of hope for individuals seeking paths to wellness.

I am thankful to God for helping me discover the "FAB FIVE" and finding complete healing from Ulcerative Colitis.

I appreciate my family, especially Mum and Sister, for supporting me throughout my journey.

And to YOU, thank you for letting me join you on your path to healing. I hope your journey is full of health, joy, and ongoing achievements—cheers to a future and the endless possibilities of wellness.

I wish you all the Best!
Lorna Hart

Appendices: Additional Tips on Supplements and Food

Appendix A; Supplementary Guide

Probiotics

Suggested Brand; [PROBIO 7. ORIGINAL-10 BILLION FRIENDLY BACTERIA)

Daily Intake: 10 to 20 billion CFUs

Tips: opt for probiotics with various strains containing Lactobacillus and Bifidobacterium species.

Flaxseed- Omega 3 Fatty Acids

Best Source: Fish oil supplements or flaxseed oil/blended grains

Daily Intake: 1,000 3,000 mg

Tips: Make sure the supplement is clean from metals and impurities.

Blackseed oil

When selecting black seed oil, it is crucial to prioritise quality. Here are some pointers for spotting a top-notch product.

1. Cold Pressed: Make sure the oil is cold pressed to retain its nutrients
2. Organic: opt for organic certified oil for pesticide levels and better overall quality.
3. Pure and Unrefined: Look for oil that's pure, unrefined, and free from any additives.

4. Dark Glass Bottle: Choose oil stored in glass bottles as they shield it from exposure and help preserve its potency.
5. Trusted Brands: Some known brands to consider are www.TheBlessed seed.com, Amazing Herbs, Kiva and Health Logics.

For Daily Use.

The recommended black seed oil dosage can differ based on your purpose and individual health conditions. Here are some general suggestions.

- For Adults: For General Health: 1 to 2 teaspoons per day.
- For Therapeutic Purposes: Up to 2 to 3 teaspoons, depending on your condition and advice from a healthcare professional.
- For Children: It's best to consult with a paediatrician. Children over five years old can start with ½ to 1 teaspoon daily.

Usage Tips.

Begin with an amount if you're new to seed oil—around half a teaspoon. Then, gradually increase the dosage based on your tolerance level until you reach the desired intake amount. Take black seed oil with food to improve absorption and avoid stomach discomfort. Mix the oil with honey or juice if you find the taste unpleasant. Blend it into a smoothie. To see results, make sure to use it over an extended period. Additionally, you can apply topically black seed oil for its skin and hair benefits by blending a drop with carrier oil such as coconut before using it on your skin.

Recommended Foods

Include in Your Diet.

- Vegetables like leafy greens, carrots, and zucchini
- Fruits such as bananas, apples (peeled) and blueberries
- Protein sources like meats, fish, eggs, and tofu

- Grains like white rice, quinoa, and gluten-free oats
- fats from olive oil, coconut oil, and avocado

Foods to Limit or Avoid.

- Dairy products include milk, cheese, and butter.
- Gluten-containing foods like wheat, barley, and rye.
- Processed foods such as packaged snacks and fast-food items
- Sugary treats like soda, candies, and pastries
- Nightshade vegetables such as tomatoes, peppers, and eggplants

Sample Meal Plan.

Start your day with a nutritious smoothie made with spinach, banana, almond milk, and flaxseed oil. For lunch, enjoy a quinoa salad topped with grilled chicken, cucumbers and olive oil dressing.

Dinner could be baked salmon served with steamed broccoli. And sweet potato. Snack on carrot sticks with hummus or apple slices. With almond butter.

Techniques for Managing Stress

- Mindfulness Meditation.
- Take 10 to 20 minutes each day to practice mindfulness meditation.
- Sit comfortably.
- Focus on your breathing.
- And gently guide your thoughts back when they stray.
- Yoga Practice.
- Engage in yoga sessions lasting 20 to 30 minutes.
- 3 to 4 times per week. Try poses such as Childs Pose,
- Cat Cow Stretch,
- or Legs Up the Wall.

- Focus on poses that promote relaxation. Keeping a journal is recommended. Share your emotions, happenings and things that bother you. Also, focus on the moments of your day.

- For relaxation, try the 4, 7, and 8 breathing techniques. Breathe in for 4 seconds, hold for 7 seconds, and exhale for 8 seconds. Repeat this cycle 4 to 5 times. Exercise Recommendations

- For low-impact activities, Experts suggest that you engage in walking for 30 minutes daily.

- Swimming three times a week

- Cycling, for 20 to 30 minutes 3 to 4 times per week

- Strength training should be done 2 to 3 times weekly, focusing on bodyweight exercises like squats, lunges, push-ups, and resistance bands. Each session should last around 20 to 30 minutes.

- Consider incorporating yoga and Tai Chi into your routine to improve flexibility and balance. Aim to practice these 2 to 3 times weekly for 20 to 30 minutes each session.

Additional Resources for Reading

"The Autoimmune Solution" by Dr. Amy Myers

"The Wahls Protocol" by Dr. Terry Wahls

"Gut and Psychology Syndrome" by Dr Natasha Campbell McBride

Support Groups

When seeking more information or support online, consider visiting websites such as the Crohn's & Colitis Foundation, The American Journal of Gastroenterology and PubMed. You can also join support groups through communities like Reddit or Facebook Groups. Attend local meetings organised by the Crohn's & Colitis Foundation.

References

https://www.neuralword.com/en/article/understanding-dietary-strategies-to-manage-colitis

COQ 10 - Ubidecarenone. https://www.5thnutrisupply.com/super-antioxidant/coq-10---ubidecarenone

Ulcerative Colitis: Symptoms, Treatment, and More (verywellhealth.com)